I0392710

Continuing Medical Education
What to do when good outcomes go bad...

Copyright 2016 Bonny P McClain
Published by Data & Donuts

Table of Contents

Prologue

I get bored easily. It was easy for me to transition to independent consultancy for a work environment aligned with my lifestyle, interests, and culture. No longer required to meet the conflicting and contrasting needs of a single healthcare stakeholder I hit the road to become proficient in the entire healthcare ecosystem.

Not too shabby for a first year out I attended the Whitehouse Conference on Aging, joined an interactive audience for Health Affairs Briefing: The Cost and Quality of Cancer Care at the National Press Club, National Health Statistics Conference, Addressing Economic Challenges in an Evolving Health Care Market sponsored by Brookings Institution, and investigative journalism invited by the BMJ to name just a few.

Over the ensuing years, I continue to attend panel discussions sponsored by International Society for Pharmacoeconomics and Outcomes Research (ISPOR), Patient-Centered Outcomes Research Institute (PCORI), National Academy of Medicine (NAM), and patient advocacy organizations. The most informative interactions are often during the Q & A when the attendees are able to challenge or expand on podium and panel discussions.

Networking and collaborating with health policy leaders, economists, and medical experts is only one side of a coin. Understanding how to report data and reach out to audiences that can benefit from research and conference findings is as important as the invitations to speak or lead break out sessions. I like the way a colleague described what I do "I'm a fan of her blog "Data and Donuts" that **explores the intersection of our interpretation of scientific data and how we communicate it, ensuring that we are both curious and intellectually honest.**"

I opted out of writing exclusively for continuing medical education for many reasons. The main reason was a potential conflict of interest for participation on advisory councils, panel discussions, and for many speaking opportunities outside of industry.

Another reason is the infrastructure that rewards conveniently finding gaps in disease states--and drug categories--with the deepest pockets. These small e-books are my way of sharing what I discover out on the road--information that you can bring back to your teams or your office.

I also believe that we need a modern framework for continuing medical education. Governing bodies and associations are vying for seats at the table to expand the role and function of educational programs in issues of policy compliance and clinical practice improvement activities.

Clinicians are heterogeneous and do not practice in a vacuum. The traditional format (epidemiology, clinical practice, guideline directed care, gaps, and educational platform to close them) may have been the best we could do prior to healthcare reform but public databases, health policy advances seeking to identify value frameworks, and health economics and outcomes research require integration of context in clinical decisions at the point of care.

The old template has limited applicability to the emerging complexities of modern medicine.

A modern list of NA inclusion:

Begin with SMART learning objectives. SMART outcome objectives measure quantifiable progress against benchmarks and specific goals supported by measurable data. I discuss how to write learning objectives in a short guide titled, The Learning Objective: Identifying appropriate metrics for improving medical education--as a refresher they stand for **S**pecific, **M**easurable, **A**chievable, **R**elevant, and **T**ime-bound.

Current practice	High-value practice
A brief disease-state background	Population relevant disease-state background—recent aggregated data
	Shared decision making
Currently available therapies	Benefits and harms of available therapies
Therapies under development	What do novel therapies add to armatorium? Cost? Efficacy? Safety?
Practice guidelines	Multi-criteria decision analysis (MCDA) Level of evidence and funding sources of current guidelines (supporting data and research)
Current practice	Longitudinal data describing medical expenditures, outcomes, and variables of interest (social determinants, demographics etc.)
Deficits in practice	Localized data and outcomes
Practice gaps	Downstream costs of therapies post-market due to adverse events
Educational needs	Patient reported outcomes stratified with clinical needs and gaps in care.

It can be confusing when evaluating clinical reports or research studies. A careful analysis should do the following:

- Exclude evidence from the current clinical trial—what is the plausibility of the different treatment effects? In Bayesian analysis we call this the "prior distribution". What do we know already?
- What support exists for the different treatment effects based only on the data in the current clinical trial? This is "likelihood".
- If you combine the "priors" and the "likelihood" we now have our statistical insights about the treatment effect—the "posterior distribution".

Here is a quote from the CME Coalition:

"The mechanisms already in place ensure that accredited/certified CME activities are designed to address clinicians' practice-relevant learning needs and practice gaps. The programs are also measured to evaluate the educational and clinical impact of the activity. Finally, they are planned and provided independent from commercial influence or other biases."

A strong lobby can only take CME so far. We need to modernize our approach to provide value in the emerging healthcare framework. We can add patient partnerships, shared-decision making (with trade-offs clearly defined), and quality of life in addition to emergent themes of relevance.

In the figure below, a variety of considerations at the private and commercial sector demonstrate where opportunities exist to balance health and social needs—often reached at the point of care. Commercial headroom describes an "effectiveness gap" or the net benefit recognized if the intervention were provided for free.

Using Multicriteria Decision Analysis to Support Research Priority Setting in Biomedical Translational Research Projects

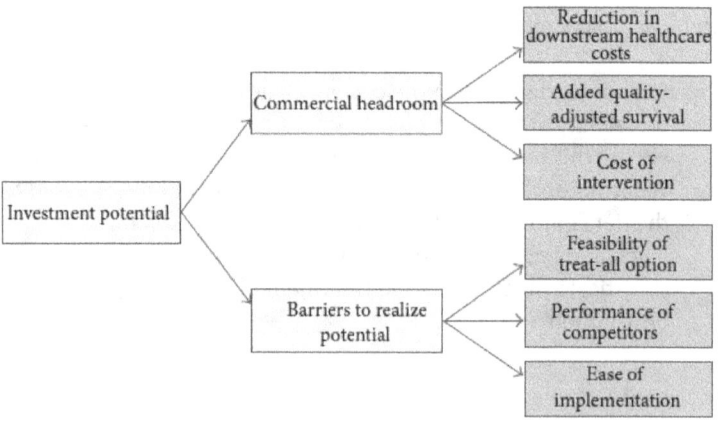

In healthcare, stakeholders are required to make trade-offs. Decisions on behaviors at the point of care aligned with the highest potential of

improving patient outcomes at a reasonable cost benefit from multicriteria decision analysis (MCDA). Clinicians are heterogeneous and do not practice in a vacuum. The old format may have been the best we could do prior to healthcare reform but public databases, health policy advances seeking to identify value frameworks, and health economics and outcomes research require integration of context in clinical decisions at the point of care.

Multicriteria decision analysis is a relatively new application for healthcare although it has existed in a variety of industries. I would recommend a review of the literature provided by organizations such as International Pharmacoeconomics (ISPOR) especially if you are interested in applying shared-decision making objectives to medical education topics.

As healthcare transitions to being truly patient focused with engagement— MCDA is needed to blend objective and subjective considerations into the treatment dialogue. Think about pragmatic clinical trials and the need to consider both randomized clinical trial findings from controlled environments to create a bridge from research to clinical care.

Over-estimated intervention benefit and under-estimated harm

Everyone is discussing patient-centricity and shared decision-making. I would suggest that for some it is a genuine objective but for many others it is a marketing tool. Once you get patients reporting the benefits of a treatment—particularly a drug about to lose patent protection—the patient advocacy groups are mobilized to market on behalf of industry behind the shadow of efficacy and true need.

Patients' Expectations of the Benefits and Harms of Treatments, Screening, and Tests A Systematic Review, published in JAMA Internal Medicine journal is informative.

> *The majority of participants overestimated intervention benefit and underestimated harm. Clinicians should discuss accurate and balanced information about intervention benefits and harms with patients, providing the opportunity to develop realistic expectations and make informed decisions.*

Think about the environment that influences these perceptions. Make a mental note about the quantity of direct to consumer advertising that reaches the population (and future client base) regarding their sex drive, cardiovascular health, diabetes, thinning hair, attention deficit, and the list goes on. This amount of marketing is being targeted to a client base that will need permission to make the purchase. Obviously you can't just limp into a store and pull a new hip off of the shelf. There are numerous episodic evaluations and financial transactions that have to be launched for any of the point of sale objectives.

There is a groundswell of interest emerging in improving adherence, patient centricity, creating and identifying value, and understanding healthcare policy and governance.

Patient engagement is pursued *with* the patient—not something we do *to* the patient.

I suggest you pick a parade and get in front. Develop content that matters and informs. Or you are going to need a shovel. A big shovel.

I suggest you read, **A Framework For Organizing And Selecting Quantitative Approaches For Benefit-Harm Assessment**

Source: *BMC Medical Research Methodology 2012*; **12**:173
http://www.biomedcentral.com/1471-2288/12/173

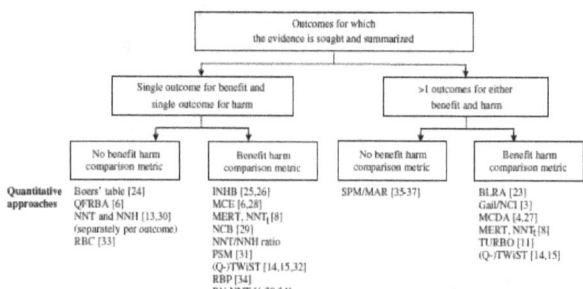

Figure 1 Key characteristics of the benefit-harm question that may guide selection of quantitative assessment for benefit-harm assessment. Abbreviations: *INHB*, Incremental net health benefit; *MCE*, Minimum clinical efficacy; *NCB*, Net Clinical Benefit; *NNT*, Number needed to treat; *NNH*, Number needed to treat for harm; *Q-Twist*, (Quality-adjusted) Time without Symptoms and Toxicity; *RBC*, Risk–benefit contour; *RV-NNT*, Relative value adjusted number needed to treat; *QFRBA*, Quantitative Framework for Risk and Benefit Assessment; *TURBO*, Transparent Uniform Risk Benefit; *BLRA*, Benefit-less-risk analysis; *PSM*, Probabilistic simulation methods; *MERT*, Minimum Target Event Risk for Treatment; *MCDA*, Multicriteria decision analysis: *RBP*, Risk–benefit plane; *SPM*, Stated preference method; *MAR*, Maximum acceptable risk.

This simple graphic is pinned on the wall in my office and it drives all the CME content I develop. I suggest you take a look and familiarize yourself with the quantitative approaches.

I tackle common topics in Improving Numeracy in Medicine and on the blog http://www.dataanddonuts.org and http://www.alzheimersdiseasethebrand.com.

The ability to quantify and qualify data to inform the evidence requires an understanding of numeracy and a willingness to dig a little deeper.

The next graphic is a simple flow sheet created to visualize different drug categories, risks/benefits, and contextualizes the findings. It is an early template for type 2 diabetes (T2D) where I added links to data and figures unique to each drug category.

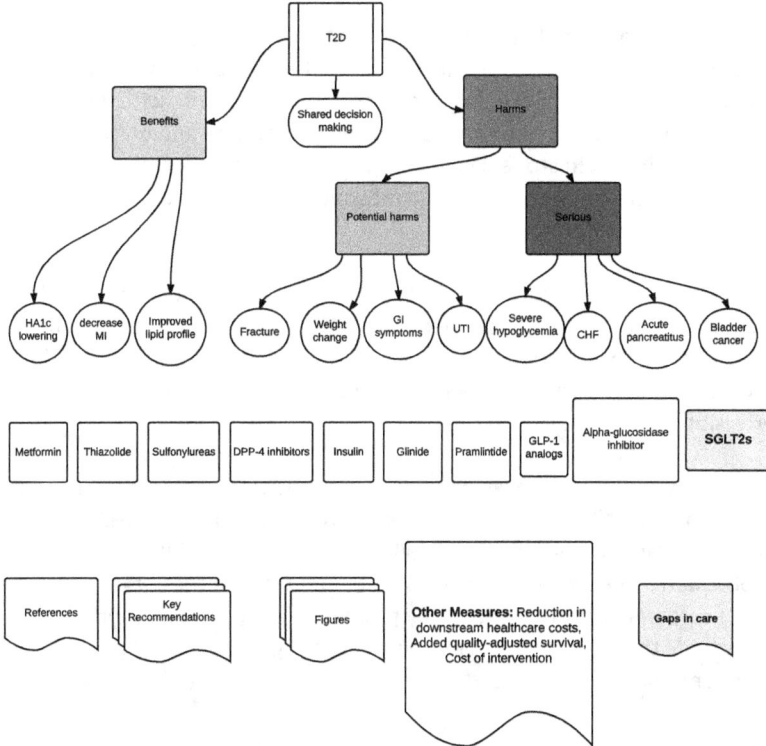

Looking for value in CME

The way we measure value is often flawed. I am not considering the squishy definition of value that provides an estimate of low- or high-value outcomes in healthcare. I am more or less referring to how we evaluate physician learning in continuing medical education. I work with data often provided post-activity once all the front-end objectives and metrics become firewalled and set in stone. Obviously not ideal but these datasets provide a systemic glimpse of persistent misconceptions in how we are evaluating learning outcomes.

Continuing medical education (CME) professionals assigned the task of working with outcomes data seek ways to describe significant patterns in informative and narrative formats. Numbers and units combine to yield accurate measurements. But what is the difference between accuracy and precision?

How many participants answered this question? How many answered the question correctly pre- and post-activity? These are all examples of accuracy. Basically, are my results aligned with the truth? It becomes problematic when we make leaps of faith and claim, if these measurements are accurate; the participants in my program clearly have learned something they didn't know before participating in my learning intervention.

> *"When you measure, you must interpret the measurement against the standard established by the tool. In the process, you put a little bit of yourself into the measurement and, for this reason; the tool you use to measure has a big impact on the result you get. The existence of a measurement, not surprisingly, means that someone actually measured it. There is a natural limit to how well I can measure objects depending on how well I can 'see' it as well as how good of a tool I am using to see it—Matt Anticole*

So far sounds pretty straightforward but what if we aren't using the right tool or aren't using the tool properly?

Accuracy vs. Precision

Now we are considering precision. If you have developed the right tool based on specificity and exactness of measurement then you now have the confidence to report your findings.

Basically you can accurately measure before and after statistics for your educational interventions and report what you find but if you want to be precise you need to switch to a more "finely incremented" tool.

What can we do to achieve this higher level of granularity? First, ask the right demographic questions, evaluate pre-existing heuristics and biases, measure exposure to ongoing education (how are clinical questions answered on a daily basis, record other CME or CE programs completed during your evaluation window), and don't be afraid to include measures that reflect a readiness to change.

Everything you create needs to be informed by a creative and aesthetic lens. Think about how usability has informed much of what we know about design or even interactivity in survey design, learning platforms, or to encourage engagement with your website or blog posts. Social media has driven us all to become more aware of the look and feel of the content we develop and I for one welcome the evolution.

In my professional work I often review and analyze CME outcomes that I did not develop or design. It might be because at the launch phase everything seems possible. Your educational program was funded, what could go wrong—full steam ahead! There is one reoccurring dilemma that I want to try and help you avoid.

Now let me qualify this by saying I know how limited CME budgets can be and how many of the steps associated with survey design or question structure may seem straightforward enough that you attempt to fly solo. That's fine too but I think I can help keep your journey safe and more importantly statistically rigorous.

I think it will be easier to appreciate the guidance if you try to appreciate the difference between a problem and an issue. Once you define a specific problem it becomes easier to create a checklist of concise issues that you have the power to resolve immediately. For example, a limited budget for statistical consulting may undermine your wish list of developing strong outcomes data (problem) but limited understanding of a data framework can be resolved with a helping hand or a reference resource (issue).

I say this with the understanding--nobody wants to be told his or her baby is ugly. I get it. But we can do better.

Many question designers rely on evaluating percent correct on a knowledge type question. Perhaps you even integrate a case study or an informative question stem followed by a list of potential decisions or answers. Outcomes data that I recently reviewed had these question types coded as either correct or incorrect. As I read on in the reports I see that the t-test or ANOVA statistical procedures were proudly cited but there is one problem. Dichotomous data is not normally distributed and these statistical procedures require the assumption that the data are normally distributed.

Inferences from your data are now invalid and do not report the findings that you had hoped for. I have encountered numerous occasions where the go-to statistical procedure was the t-test (or ANOVA) without consideration of whether it is actually the correct test to use.

When I design survey instruments I prefer a ranking or Likert approach but again this introduces additional statistical complexity. Why Likert? In medicine there is rarely a wrong or right question that can be applied to all patients. Because of nuances of the healing arts I try to avoid labeling and therefore analyzing a response as either correct or incorrect. The most useful advice I can recommend when you are designing these elements with limited resources--clarify what you intend to do with your data.

If you are able to rank responses, the answers are now informative. If you analyze results on a Likert scale and notice a score of 4 for multiple responses you may infer similar or equivalent measures. Unfortunately this may yield false equivalence if you assume a score of "4" always means the same thing but the respondent didn't intend for that interpretation.

The gold standard for statistical analyses would be to assign 100 points total and ask respondents to assign points to their responses.

If you are interested in showing that scores differ when considering different groups of participants (primary care physician vs. specialists), you may treat your scores as numeric values, provided they fulfill usual assumptions about variance (or shape) and sample size.

If instead you are interested in highlighting how response patterns vary across subgroups, then you should consider item scores as discrete choice among a set of answer options and look for log-linear modeling, ordinal logistic regression, item-response models or any other statistical model that allows us to cope with polytomous items vs. dichotomous.

Big data or the right data?

The majority of us reading these words speak English as a primary language. Clearly that statistic is going to be changing in the near future but for the most part, we will be able to communicate clearly and effectively with a common dialect and lexicon of understanding.

Underlying this ability to share thoughts and insights will be a new mother tongue--statistics. We are awash in big data and the ability to measure our health metrics, entertainment preferences, consumer habits, and overall personal and professional outcomes will be unparalleled. Troubling to those of us in the medical space, either as writers, researchers, practitioners, or journalists is the lack of understanding of what these data points reveal.

In a recent publication, Bernard Marr also makes the important distinction between Big data and Smart data. People within the medical education sphere pinball between sample size, effect size, p-values, confidence intervals; you name it, trying to find the magic metric for claiming an ever shrinking slice of the pharmaceutical-industry stakeholder pie. I collaborate with teams blending a weird combination of skills firewalled behind verticals. A team "owns" the actual query that generates the data, another the actual numbers, analytics, reporting, etc.

What results is a confusion of "tongues" not unlike the fabled tower of babel. There is a lack of understanding how these specific skills should harmonize to inform. You may recall a time in a far away land when showing up with data made you credible. "Oh look there is data to support my view or assertion"...not too long after, the head scratching and arched eyebrows commenced. We are duped by data every single day. Look at the latest research findings from peer-reviewed journals. It is important to build teams that contribute rigor, insight, and findings of meaningful data. Analysis doesn't begin after the data is gathered my friends. It begins with a question.

I have difficulty separating educational outcomes from actual health outcomes. Continuing medical education needs to evoke a data driven framework and in my opinion, measuring the utility of misguided educational objectives is a waste of time.

Data is often manipulated to demonstrate a weak benefit for participants in an educational program. Granted this is just my experience but here is how CME companies typically approach me:

Please write gap statements about disease x. Can you focus on this category of drugs? What? Wait. Let me explain why this never works out. Or why it never works out if the true objective is to improve patient outcomes and to partner with clinicians to provide value-based care.

Utilization-Focused Evaluation (UFE) developed by Michael Quinn Patton, states -- evaluations should be judged on usefulness to intended users. A primary goal in CME is to encourage professionals to participate in evaluations. How much time do you dedicate to planning and conducting evaluations and metrics aligned with how clinicians practice medicine.

UFE suggests that we clearly identify and engage intended users to guide decisions made about the evaluation process. In your role as an evaluator the habit of making decisions independently of your participants may be a hard habit to break but your role is to facilitate decision making for the clinicians that will use findings of the evaluation.

The 17 Step UFE Framework can be customized for therapeutic categories but here are the general principles for consideration. The bolded emphasis is mine and highlights the framework components I adapt for the majority of programs.

- Assess and build program and organizational readiness for utilization-focused evaluation
- **Assess and enhance evaluator readiness and competence to undertake a utilization-focused evaluation**
- Identify, organize, and engage primary intended users: the personal factor
- **Situation analysis conducted jointly with primary intended users**
- Identify and prioritize primary intended uses by determining priority purposes
- Consider and build in process uses if and as appropriate
- **Focus priority evaluation questions**
- **Check that fundamental areas for evaluation inquiry are being adequately addressed: implementation, outcomes, and attribution questions**
- **Determine what intervention model or theory of change is being evaluated**
- Negotiate appropriate methods to generate credible findings that support intended use by intended users
- **Make sure intended users understand potential methods controversies and their implications**
- Simulate use of findings: evaluation's equivalent of a dress rehearsal
- Gather data with ongoing attention to use
- **Organize and present the data for interpretation and use by primary intended users: analysis, interpretation, judgment, and recommendations**
- Prepare an evaluation report to facilitate use and disseminate significant findings to expand influence
- **Follow up with primary intended users to facilitate and enhance use**
- **Meta-evaluation of use: be accountable, learn, and improve**

Algorithms—bad and good

For better or worse we are transitioning into a data driven society. Mathematical patterns in data that are repetitive often yield algorithms. Kevin Slavin, in a popular Ted Talk, "How Algorithms Shape our World" argues that they acquire the sensibility of truth—they ossify and become real--often to the detriment of the details that generate them. Three aspects of algorithmic ordering of information have provoked particular scrutiny. The data used may be inaccurate or inappropriate. Algorithmic modeling may be biased or limited. And the uses of algorithms are still opaque in many critical sectors.

To appreciate the power of algorithms think of the resources committed to Spread Networks--"At 825 miles and 13.3 milliseconds, Spread's circuit shaves 100 miles and 3 milliseconds off of the previous route of lowest latency, engineer-talk for length of delay."

The genesis of an algorithm stems from the desire to break a BIG thing into many little parts. But when we relinquish control to expediency and efficiency we lose the ability to react in real time to what is now relatively automated. Think of Wall Street and the black box that hunts for electronic communications--moving a million shares through the market. Or the last economic crash. Nobody controlled the crash—only the monitor with a red button that said, "stop".

We are writing things that we can no longer understand or separate into components to inform behavior. We lost the sense of what is happening. Unfortunately algorithms are often in conflict with human oversight. Think of the automation strategies of Amazon and Netflix. These algorithms can go out of control and list books like The Making a Fly: The Genetics of Animal Design for $23,698,655.93.

Netflix and Pragmatic Chaos searched for a piece of code 10% more efficient than the current movie recommendation algorithm--and won a cool million in the process. Algorithms are evolving from being a metaphor to actual prophecy. I am thinking that we need to take a few gigantic steps backward. I figure--based on estimates derived on Google and by physician leaders there are literally thousands of guidelines for managing the health of patients. Many of them contradict the status quo and each other; few recommend less care or more deliberate watchful waiting.

The Guidelines International Network database currently contains more than 3,700 clinical practice guidelines from 39 countries. Additionally, there are nearly 2,700 guidelines in the National Guidelines Clearinghouse (NGC), part of the Agency for Healthcare Research and Quality (AHRQ). Because of the large number of clinical practice guidelines available, guideline users, including practitioners, find it challenging to determine which guidelines are of high quality. -

On the other extreme, there is an important area of medicine that is still lacking in treatment-based expert review or consensus guidelines. I will write more in another post but I thought it interesting that an important consideration for patients undergoing chemotherapeutic regimens is rarely discussed in public forums.

Examples

The first priority for developing impactful medical education includes the ability to contextualize healthcare challenges within the system at large and funnel towards a specific therapeutic area. An understanding of the evolving healthcare ecosystem is required to level-set the content. Here is a high-level review of what I might consider when writing content in an educational framework.

I am intentionally not including a recipe but a few ideas to consider. I still offer free 15 minute consultations for your content planning—send me an email and we can schedule.

In the modern healthcare dynamic there are thousands of healthcare guidelines to direct model care and improved patient outcomes. In that vast number there are certainly conflicting reports and stakeholder influence to add to the confusion.

Can we make a difference in designing content?

Listening to experts discuss cholesterol you often hear the phrase LDL hypothesis. Research appears to weaken earlier claims of LDL as a metric linked to cardiovascular outcomes. The research about VLDL or small particle cholesterol is evolving to be the component of cholesterol linked to poor outcomes. The next question should be why are statins still being prescribed. Why indeed...

So how do we structure a discussion around cholesterol? I want to use as a framework, the PCSK9 Inhibitors for Treatment of High Cholesterol: Effectiveness, Value, and Value- Based Price Benchmarks http://cepac.icer-review.org/adaptations/cholesterol/. Technology assessments are informative and complicated to write--trust me on this one. The Institute for Clinical and Economic Review (ICER) completed this one fairly recently so I think it colors this discussion in an important way. The consideration of scientific evidence should drive all content.

A lot of information to consider I know. Writing potential learning objectives that are actionable, measurable, and relevant often take the "easy" way out.

The majority of learning objectives floating around the Internet don't seem up to the heavy lifting required to be of service to healthcare provider learners at the point of care. What do you think?

- Train other healthcare providers to convey to patients their LDL cholesterol levels and what they should be
- Demonstrate the link of LDL cholesterol to the prospect of having a heart attack or stroke.
- Compare and contrast differences between various dyslipidemia guidelines and recommendations (ACC/AHA vs. NLA vs. AACE) for atherosclerotic cardiovascular disease (ASCVD) prevention in terms of lipid goals, evidence-base, risk calculators, and non-statin therapies.
- Examine the scientific rationale behind targeting specific lipoprotein levels for LDL-C, non-HDL-C, Apo B, triglycerides, and HDL-C to reduce cardiovascular risk and review the evidence for the use of combination pharmacologic therapy to effectively treat dyslipidemia.
- Explore newly recognized pathways in lipid metabolism and examine the role of CETP inhibition in lipid disorders.
- Review the efficacy and safety profiles of CETP inhibitors currently in clinical development to elucidate potential implications for future practice.

- Summarize current guideline recommended strategies for the treatment of hypercholesterolemia in adults to reduce atherosclerotic cardiovascular risk.
- Identify the pathophysiologic roles of apolipoprotein B, PCSK9, and microsomal triglyceride transfer proteins in regulating serum LDL-cholesterol.

- Assess current data and potential role of novel and emerging cholesterol-lowering agents in patients with hypercholesterolemia who are intolerant to statins or require additional LDL-C reduction.

There are many variables to consider when identifying metrics for predicting adverse cardiac events. I believe evidence demonstrates LDL-P (or apoB) as best predictor of adverse cardiac events documented repeatedly in every major cardiovascular risk study. But what about LDL you might be thinking? There are studies that demonstrate LDL as a good predictor of adverse cardiac events but dig a little deeper and only when concordant with LDL-P; otherwise it is a poor predictor of risk.

You need to follow reliable sources of information. I recommend **theBMJ** http://www.bmj.com/theBMJ for many reasons but their tag line has become a professional heuristic—**answering questions, and questioning answers.**

When you read CME learning objectives written within your team or across the Internet—evaluate them. And then, do better.

- Integrate guidelines *(which ones?)* and treatment targets (for what patient populations?) into patient-centric *(does this mean shared-decision making?)* cholesterol management plans
- Identify and address limitations *(Efficacy? Efficiency? Cost? Patient outcomes?)* of statin therapy *(drug specific? class of drugs specific? Comorbidities?)* in achieving treatment targets (in what patient populations?)
- Describe mechanisms-of-action of emerging hypercholesterolemia agents based on targets in lipoprotein synthesis, transport, and regulation *(this is actually at least 3 different learning objectives, what about triglycerides? --what about genetic susceptibility?)*
- Outline clinical trial data on the efficacy and safety of novel agents for lowering LDL cholesterol *(all the clinical trial data? what about other risk factors associated with disease? Non-inferiority trials? Placebo trials? Lifestyle intervention trials?)*
- Review the fundamental role of HDL-C in atherosclerosis development, as well as its potential as a therapeutic target through CETP inhibition *(education on clinical surrogate end-points?)*
- **Discuss the latest data available on PCSK9 inhibition as a potential LDL-C–lowering strategy (stratify the data for RCT? Limitations of meta-analyses)**

Critically evaluate the pros and cons of the current ACC/AHA and NLA cholesterol guidelines *(what about other guidelines? NICE? ICSI? AACE? -- Are they asking you to review the data?)*

Follow organizations for context and training opportunities

Everyone is talking about big data. We create data but what can we learn about the data we are already collecting? Do you know what are actually "noise" and what is actually informing and guiding future activities? How can you operationalize and scale your data to create value?

The Institute for Clinical and Economic Review (ICER) is an independent non-profit research organization that evaluates medical evidence and convenes public deliberative bodies to help stakeholders interpret and apply evidence to improve patient outcomes and control costs. ICER receives funding from government grants, non-profit foundations, health plans, provider groups, and health industry manufacturers. Through all its work, ICER seeks to help create a future in which collaborative efforts to move evidence into action provide the foundation for a more effective, efficient, and just health care system. More information about ICER is available at http://www.icer- review.org

---

Institute for Clinical and Economic Review (ICER) Action Guide includes key recommendations and resources to help stakeholders apply evidence to guidance to practice and policy. http://cepac.icer-review.org/wp-content/uploads/2015/04/PCSK9-Action-Guide-for-Clinicians-and-Policy-Makers1.pdf

The New England Comparative Effectiveness Public Advisory Council (CEPAC) is an independent, regional body of practicing physicians, methodological experts, and leaders in patient advocacy and engagement that provides objective, independent guidance on the application of medical evidence to clinical practice and payer policy decisions across New England.

Read the documents and see what you think. Here is a quote from the section on Harms.

> *Nearly all studies have less than 6 months of follow-up data, but results from individual studies and from the Navarese meta-analysis have found that PCSK9 drugs are very well tolerated; there have been no findings suggestive of significant increases in adverse event rates. There are more injection site reactions, which may lead to slightly higher rates of drug discontinuation compared to the control group. There is a slight excess of neurocognitive events with PCSK9 inhibitors, but the results are not statistically significant. There is also a trend towards more myalgias in the PCSK9 treated participants, but this is balanced by a statistically significant reduction in the number of participants with elevations in the muscle enzyme creatine kinase (CK). Detailed adverse event-rate data are provided in the full report.*

This is utter nonsense. Less than 6 months of follow-up data is not enough data. Period. Phrases like "very well-tolerated" do not have a place in a medical report. How does a physician quantify "very-well tolerated" at the point of care? "No findings suggestive of **significant increases** in adverse event rates". When discussing adverse events, referring to increases as significant is sloppy. Statistically or clinically? Slightly higher rates of drug discontinuation?

Take the time to understand numeracy and to **question answers**.

Perhaps your team has uneven skills and requires foundational learning within your specific industry or vertical. Your statistical and data analyses solutions are relevant.

Welcome to the value economy. You either are sighing, "Its about time" or your are concerned about your bottom line. My assumption is that you are looking for a lifeline in navigating how to align communication strategies, performance metrics, and disease state data (numeracy) with business objectives.

The business objectives might be educational programs for healthcare providers, informative articles, or more of an understanding of our evolving healthcare ecosystem.

One-on-one conversations with industry leaders reveal the common concern. It is time we focus on the goal. Improving our healthcare system, quality of care, and most importantly--patient outcomes that reflect the values and needs of shared-decision makers--the patient—should be the common goal.

Picture the physician at the point of care. Now re-envision your skills, awareness, and numeracy. The partnership is irrefutable.

What should we do now?

There is also a disconnect between what doctors want in medical education and what they are being provided. For example, Family Medicine practitioners desperately need resources to help their patients BEFORE they are diagnosed with chronic disease.

1. Utilization of ancillary services (diabetic counseling for diet, exercise regimens for weight loss and other therapeutic lifestyle changes for comorbid disease) is not applied routinely in caring for the diabetic patient despite guideline recommendations advocating these elements. This is due to lack of time, resource access and financial coverage.

2. Screening for, and treatment of, other comorbid conditions (hypertension, dyslipidemia) do not occur consistently.

3. Physicians do not take advantage of opportunities for managing at risk populations prior to the onset of clinical diabetes.

4. Patient registries and group medical appointments to identify and manage cohorts of diabetic patients within practices are still underutilized, despite government and insurer incentives to institute these.
But what do many CME stakeholders request? Data to support treating numbers, pharmaceuticals to tighten glycemic control, and other cost drivers of healthcare.

###

Connect with me:

Twitter: http://twitter.com/graphemeconsult or
http://twitter.com/dataanddonuts

Subscribe to my blog:
http://www.dataanddonuts.org

http://www.alzheimersdiseasethebrand.com

Books available at Amazon and your favorite retailer
http://www.amazon.com/Bonny-P-McClain/e/B00J0M10OY

Improving Numeracy in Medicine
Medical Writing For Smart People
The Learning Objective
5 Sources for the Right Healthcare Data
Write Better Surveys. Period
Blueprint for a Scalable Health Data Strategy (Pre-order discounts)

Resources

http://betterevaluation.org/plan/approach/utilization_focused_evaluation

http://www.ispor.org/GuidelinesIndex/

http://www.ghdonline.org/uploads/learning_before_leaping.pdf

How algorithms shape our world.
https://www.ted.com/talks/kevin_slavin_how_algorithms_shape_our_world?language=en

http://cepac.icer-review.org/wp-content/uploads/2015/04/PCSK9-Action-Guide-for-Clinicians-and-Policy-Makers1.pdf